Secrets
Of
Aging

Staying Young and Healthy Made Easy

RON KNESS

ISBN-13: 978-1542591201

ISBN-10: 1542591201

Contents

Disclaimer

We hope you enjoy reading our report however we do suggest you read our disclaimer. All the material written in this report is provided for informational purposes only and is general in nature.

Every person is a unique individual and what has worked for some, or even many, may not work for you. Any information perceived as advice by must be considered in light of your own particular set of circumstances.

The author or person sharing this information does not assume any responsibility for the accuracy or outcome of your use of the content.

Every attempt has been made to provide well researched and up to date content at the time of writing. Now all the legalities have been taken care of, please enjoy the content.

Introduction

Welcome to our flagship product of my anti-aging website https://secretsofaging.net. If you have not yet got our free report: **Turning 50 – Congratulations Ladies, Your Life Has Just Begun**, be sure to do it from here: https://secretsofaging.net/start-here/.

We all age, and at one time or another, wish we didn't. In the majority of cases, your health, fitness, vitality and resistance to disease and infirmity comes down to your own inputs. Like any system, garbage in – garbage out.

Probably the greatest single realization that anyone facing fears of aging can embrace, is that many of the problems attributed to aging are not inevitable, or at least that the degree is not absolute.

Anti-aging involves undertaking actions that have been shown to reduce and even reverse signs and symptoms normally associated with growing older. Some of these signs are visible, others are more internal and hidden. They can be physical, mental or emotional.

Tried and tested methods exist for overcoming and dealing with these changes and also for accepting and coming to terms with them. Choose the methods that best suit your circumstances, ability and willingness. Create a toolbox of coping behaviors and habits that will help you look forward to every new day.

We have the power within us to make changes to different aspects of our lives to bring about improvements to our quality of life, now and in the future. These changes may be small initially, but can be built upon and their effects will lead to other, bigger, better changes.

The Evolution of Your Anti-Aging Plans

Good health isn't static throughout our lives. It changes. Our bodies become different and our health needs alter continually. Not just our physical health, but also our mental well-being.

Aging encompasses so much more than whatever wrinkles you see on your face. It's more than age spots or aches and pains that you feel over time. It's a total mind and body process – inside and out.

From the day we are born we start aging. In our formative years, it's up to our parents to help us prevent faster aging. For example, they choose our foods and put sunscreen on our bodies before a day at the beach.

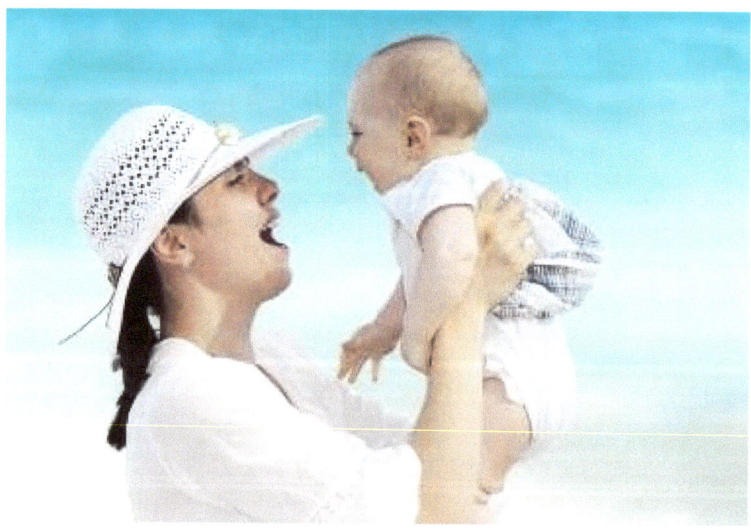

But once we reach our teen years, the responsibilities shift to us and from that point on, we should enact a self-care routine that helps us maintain our youth as long as possible.

Anti-Aging in Your Teens

It's so hard to think about anti-aging regimens when we're teenagers. After all, our bodies and minds are fit and healthy at this age. Skin is taut - and aside from acne, there are no age spots or wrinkles to be concerned with.

Still, some girls and boys in this age group *are* being educated about the aging process, so they're able to make immediate changes that help them stay younger, longer.

In your teens, you want to do everything you can to:

- Protect your skin from sun damage
- Max out your mental capabilities
- Exercise your body by pushing it to its (safe) limits
- Cater to your sleep needs
- Feed your body the nutrients it needs to thrive
- Learn how to achieve happiness and stress relief on demand

The earlier these habits are adopted, the easier it will be to utilize them in your later years. This is a time when you probably won't have trouble sleeping or finding the energy you need to accomplish your to do list.

But unfortunately, it's also a time when we're lazy about anti-aging behaviors. We go to sleep with makeup on, stay up until all hours of the night and run on fumes, lay out in the sun wearing baby oil instead of sunscreen, and so on.

Educating yourself is half the battle. Taking the needed steps to protect your youthful appearance and energy is the second – and the most important - part of your battle.

Anti-Aging in Your 20s

In our twenties, we start to recognize that time marches on. In our early twenties, we're still enjoying some of the teenaged perks we had before – but later in our twenties, we start to realize that our skin is changing, our bodies are evolving – and we're suddenly alert to those differences.

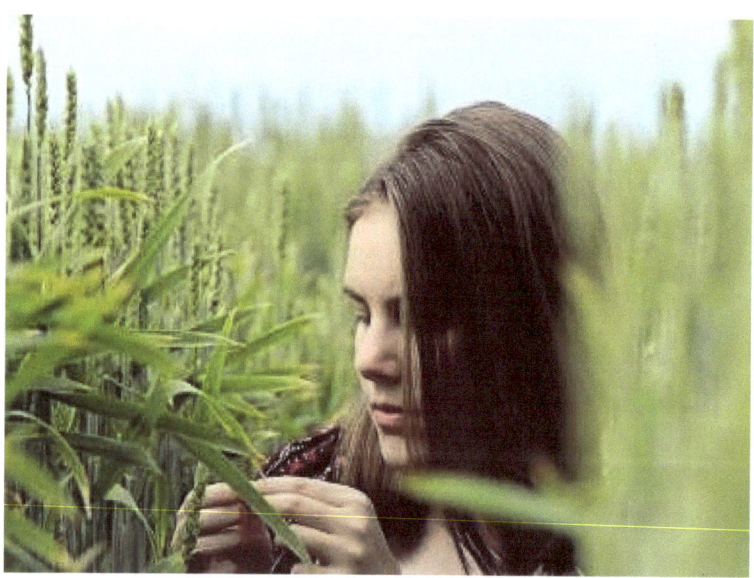

This is when you should really try to kick those awful habits you adopted in your late teens, early 20s – like smoking because you thought it would look cool, but you now realize only hurts your health (and beauty).

In your twenties, you might start seeing changes in your skin from your teen years. If you're working in your career, you also might start realizing you can't keep up with the teen and early 20s crowd like you once did – partying until 3 AM and up at 5 to go to work.

This is the decade when you wake up and start feeling – both physically and mentally – like you're not a kid anymore. It's time to start preparing for your adult years with internal and external solutions.

Anti-Aging in Your 30s

The thirties are when men and women alike sound off alarm bells in their heads about the aging process. The first real signs of aging begin to show up – your first gray hair, your first fine line around the eyes.

It's enough to send a panic through your body.

If you're a parent, then chances are you're feeling exhausted – whether it's because you're chasing toddlers around or because your body is aging faster than it should be.

This is the decade where you need to take back control. You're still young enough to be filled to the brim with energy if you approach it right – but you're old enough to understand that you can't stop time, so the self-care is imperative for you.

Anti-Aging in Your 40s

When you reach your 40th birthday, you're officially known as being "over the hill."

Everything is downhill from this point on – unless it's not! You're the only one who can determine that.

It's at this age that the signs of aging truly show up in some way, shape or form. It might be crow's feet or sagging skin that you can't seem to battle any more. Sometimes it's weight gain and depression.

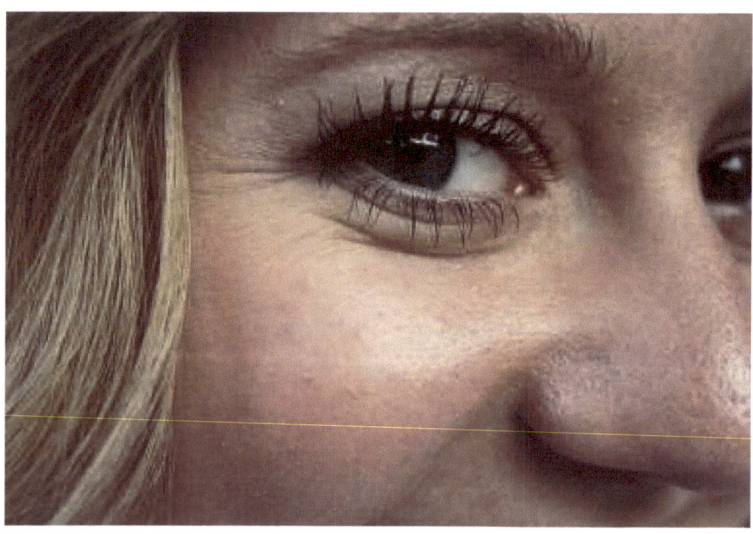

The key to fighting back against the aging process in your 40s is to adopt a regimen that suits your age.

You can't try to be more youthful by using products and strategies meant for a 20-something but you can certainly take effective steps to delay the visible and hidden effects of aging.

Anti-Aging in Your 50s and Beyond

For those who get past their 'over the hill' stage and embrace the aging process, it doesn't mean you have to neglect your body or mind – it simply means you age gracefully with beauty and poise, nurturing your skin, your physical health and your mental wellbeing the way a mother cares for her child.

It's never too late to turn back the clock. Whether you're 55 or 85, there are ways you can slow down the aging process, even reversing it in some instances.

While there's no magical fountain of youth you can jump into – there are smart, strategic steps you can take to nourish your mind and body through these years in a way that brings happiness to you.

We're going to look at an internal and external plan of attack for battling the aging process. From the foods you eat to the way you handle stress and anxiety – everything you do can have an impact on how old you look and feel.

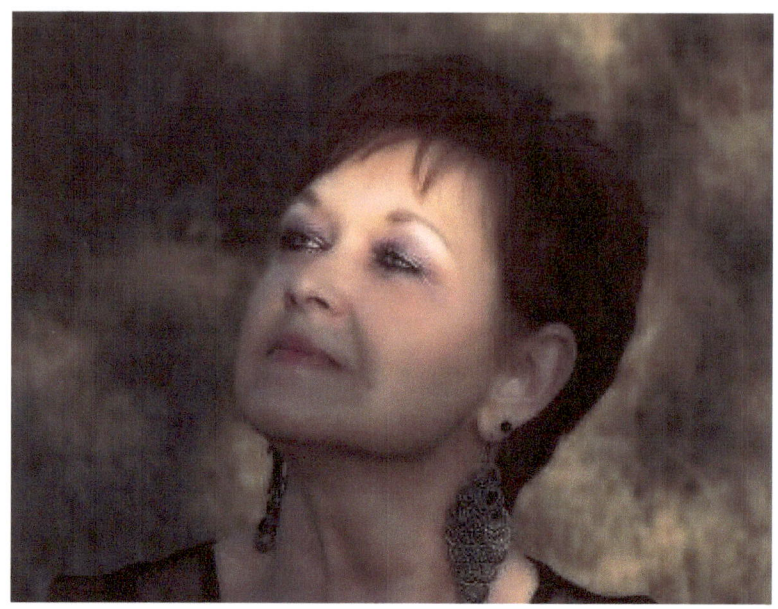

Analyzing Your Anti-Aging Needs

Before you can start treating your body with the care it deserves and craves, you have to know where it stands. Most people looking into anti-aging are already seeing or feeling symptoms of growing older – because that's when we tend to take action.

In order to get a complete picture of what needs to be done, you should get a snapshot of what's happening internally and externally.

Get Your Doctor to Conduct a Complete Health Panel

Sometimes a simple tweak of your vitamins and minerals or other health inputs can help you turn back the clock and regain some of your youthful energy and beauty.

At your next checkup, or even before, ask for a full health panel that shows any deficiencies in things like:

- Estrogen or Testosterone
- Vitamin D
- B vitamins…etc.

You want to know what your other readings are for cholesterol, triglycerides, and glucose. Knowing what diseases or risks you're at right now will help you address them so that you feel better on a regular basis from now on.

Something as simple as a vitamin D deficiency, which is very prevalent in today's world, can cause a great deal of fatigue.

You can also experience more instances of colds and flu, weakness in your muscles, depression, cancer and more.

When you get your results back, it's important that you study the range of normal. If a stat says that normal falls between 300-900, and your number is right at 300, then you might want to boost it with a supplement.

You want to recheck your health stats over time to see how things are progressing. Take note of how you look and feel as your deficiencies are cured through supplements – has it made things better?

How Do Your Looks Stack Up to Previous Years?

You have to take a cold, hard look in the mirror and be honest with yourself about how your body has held up (or not). It's okay to be concerned about beauty – not everything has to be health related.

Looking good helps us to feel good about ourselves, and that's important to our state of mind, which will subsequently affect our physical wellbeing. It doesn't mean you have to go to extremes – it just means you can start making an effort to reverse the damage that's been done from the aging process.

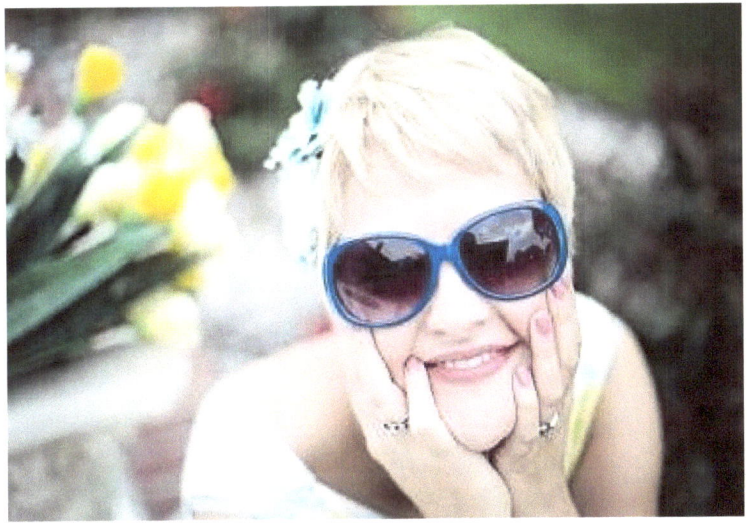

Make notes to yourself about how you look now compared to ten or fifteen years ago.

- Has your hair started to turn gray?

- Do you see age spots on your face or hands?

- Are fine lines (or deep wrinkles) showing up around your eyes and/or mouth?

- Is your skin sagging on your body?

- Has it been a while since you shopped for new clothes, got an updated haircut or started doing your makeup differently?
- Have you started gaining weight and it's not as easy to get rid of it?

These are all signs of aging that have to do with your beauty and self-confidence. Be honest with yourself and that way, you can make a plan to fix whatever is bothering you over the coming months and years.

What Physical Feelings Are Causing You to Feel Older?

Physically, you might start to show signs of aging, too. This is different from your physical *appearance* because it can impede your mobility and make daily life torturous.

When you start thinking about physical wear and tear, don't bother trying to put a label of "normal" on a physical feeling that you have. These signs of aging can be reversible, so you want to take all conditions and address them as if they are temporary.

- Are you feeling aches and pains when you move around?

- Are you sleeping better, worse or the same?

- Has your eyesight worsened?

- Do you not hear as well as you once did (hint: do people have to repeat things to you or ask you to turn down the TV?)

Don't ever tell yourself that having trouble getting up off your chair or walking longer periods of time are normal. You don't have to accept that way of life – you can change it.

Is Your Mental Well-Being Putting You in Jeopardy?

Your mental health is just as important as your physical well-being, actually more so. You need to feel good emotionally, and sometimes as we grow older, we start feeling more depressed.

- Do you find yourself feeling lonely?

- Do you have more anxiety now than in previous years?

- Do you focus on regrets that you have for things you have or haven't done in life?

There are some physical ailments that are correlated to aging that actually cause some of these symptoms, so it's vital that you be honest about your emotions and then see if there's a physical reason for them.

Your thyroid might be acting up, causing irritability and depression. Or it could be diabetes. Hormone levels can flare up or decrease, causing a change in your mood.

Even if there's not a physical health reason, then you can get the tools and strategies you need to start feeling better. No one should have to live a life where their enjoyment of daily existence is diminished by depression.

Once you've taken an honest look at where you stand physically and mentally with your body and mind, it will be time for you to choose and implement an anti-aging regimen that suits you.

Don't just pick a cookie cutter regimen that someone else advises. No two people are alike, so your needs will be different to your relatives, friends and coworkers – who mean well, but aren't in your shoes.

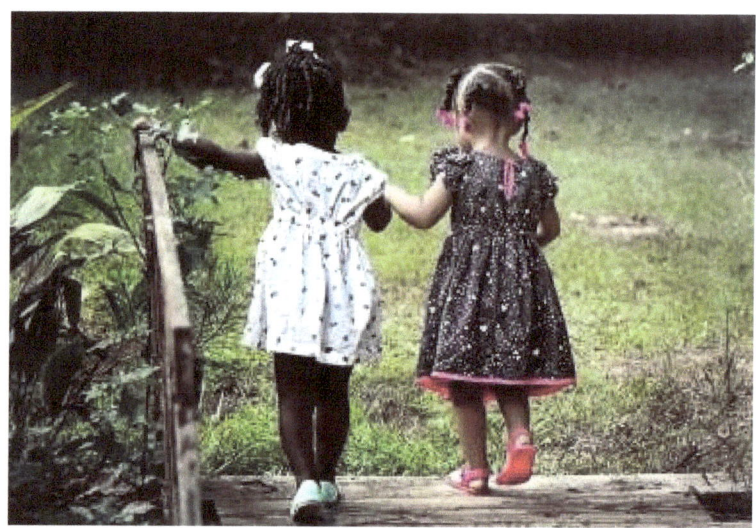

Energize Your Body and Mind

The body and mind are like *yin* and *yang* – they go together to create the person you are. When your body isn't energized, your mind becomes sluggish and vice versa.

When you're young, it seems as if you're always active and motivated, but as you age, you may need to do more to energize your body and mind. Your diet and lifestyle habits should reflect a healthy routine that will keep you looking and feeling young.

Sleep Deprivation Fast Forwards Your Aging Process

Sleep deprivation has been studied for many years as a possible detriment to graceful aging. A study conducted in July of 2013 indicates that lack of sleep can directly interfere with cognitive and memory issues of the brain.

Some types of memory tasks are more affected by lack of sleep than others. Recognition of faces is relatively unaffected by sleep deprivation whereas performing simple forms of math may be greatly affected.

Glucose tolerance and the proper functioning of the endocrine system may drastically change with sleep deprivation, accelerating age-related maladies such as hypertension, obesity, diabetes and memory loss.

Skin is also affected by sleep deprivation, states a study commissioned by the cosmetic giant, Estee Lauder and performed by scientists and physicians at University Hospitals Case Medical Center.

This team assessed those who slept well versus those who were constantly deprived of sleep and the outcome was increased signs of skin aging on the sleep-deprived group.

Lack of sleep will make almost anyone - no matter what age - feel tired. Feeling tired can cause you to perform at much less than your very best and will cause the immune system, skin, memory and cognitive abilities to mimic and exacerbate the aging process.

How much sleep you should strive for depends on your age, health and lifestyle. There's a wide spectrum of sleep needs as we age. For example, a newborn requires 12 to 18 hours of sleep per day, whereas most adults only require 7 to 9 hours per day.

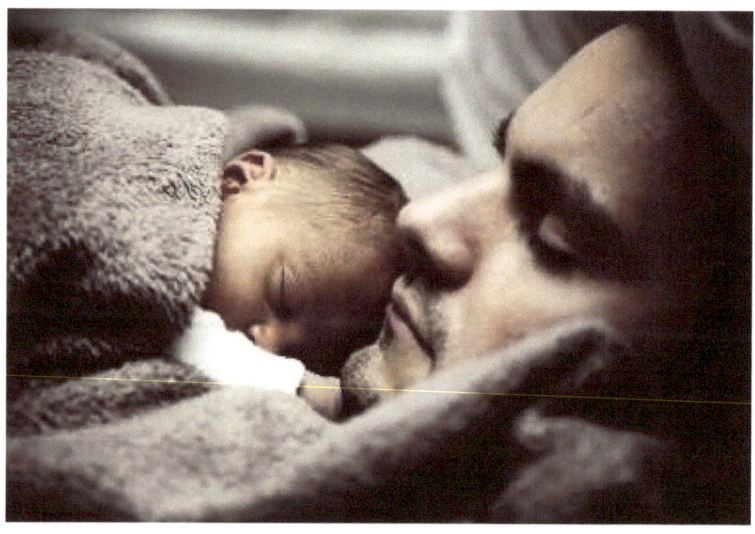

Aside from the scientific spectrum of sleep based on age, there are also other factors involving your health and lifestyle.

So, there's no magic number involved in getting enough sleep. It's based mostly on the individual. Some people feel great after sleeping seven or eight hours per night while others in the same age group may need nine hours to lead a happy and productive lifestyle.

Work schedules and amount of stress in your life also affect your sleep needs. If you're under a great deal of stress you may require more sleep for your body to experience optimal performance.

You may not be getting enough sleep if you have a sleep deficit – which is lost sleep because of illness, sudden awakenings such as for a child, an environmental factor or other reason.

If you're experiencing a sleep deficit, you may need to catch up by taking a long nap or by doing something you enjoy that is restful for the mind and body. It's also helpful to create a helpful sleep regimen that includes the following:

- Establish a relaxing routine before you go to bed such as meditation, reading, a hot bath or listening to music.

- Go to bed at the same time every day to establish consistency.

- Commit to regular exercise – but not before you go to bed.

- Be sure your sleep environment is sleep-oriented (quiet, comfy, dark and cool).

- Mattresses, pillows and other bedding needs should be soft and comfortable.

- Avoid eating for 2 to 3 hours before bedtime. Also, quit smoking and avoid alcohol and caffeine. As well as affecting sleep, these three markedly affect the body's hydration and contribute to the effects and symptoms of aging.

- Make your bedroom your sleep haven. Avoid reading, watching television or working in your bed.

A healthy amount of sleep can give you a healthier lifestyle. To find out the healthiest sleep path for you, keep track of how you react to various amounts of sleep, paying close attention to thoughts, moods, stress and energy levels after a good night's sleep or a bad night.

There are proven natural ways to combat sleep deprivation, such as exercise. Aerobic exercise releases the much-needed endorphins in your brain to relieve the stress and anxiety often associated with a poor night's sleep.

A nutritional diet is also a natural way to promote restful sleep. Studies show that those who don't sleep well at night often snack on high calorie foods during the day and are more susceptible to obesity.

Bingeing on certain foods and overeating is often due to an absence of energy from a poor night's sleep. A nutritional regimen will not only help you get a good night's sleep – it will also provide energy throughout the day and help further stave off the signs of aging.

Nutritional Regimen to Give You Extra Energy

Feeling sluggish and lacking the energy to do the things you want to do is associated with the aging process. But, it doesn't have to be that way. Adopting a good nutritional regimen at any age can give you the extra energy you need to be healthy and vital.

Removing such food items as caffeine, sodas and chocolate during the afternoon hours can help increase your energy levels. A light dinner, eaten a few hours before you go to bed may also help.

Heartburn and indigestion may keep you from getting a good night's sleep if you eat spicy or calorie-laden foods as your last meal of the day. Replacing the bad foods you usually eat with healthy ones will revitalize your energy level.

Understanding how energy works in your body will help you see how fueling the body for maximum energy can improve your ability to stay young by providing the means for moving more freely and staying alert.

The first rule of thermodynamics is that you cannot create energy. It must be converted from one type to another.

Chemical energy (adenosine triphosphate or ATP) is what the body uses for energy -- and that is solely manufactured by the body.

There are three types of body chemicals that convert to energy – carbohydrates, fats and proteins. These chemicals are turned into calories, which make up the heat we receive from food energy.

Some foods provide quick energy and others provide long-term energy. Don't think that foods high in calories will keep you energetic for the long-term. Simple carbs and sugars that provide energy in excess of what you can immediately use are most readily turned into body fat, and will cause you to feel even less energetic than before.

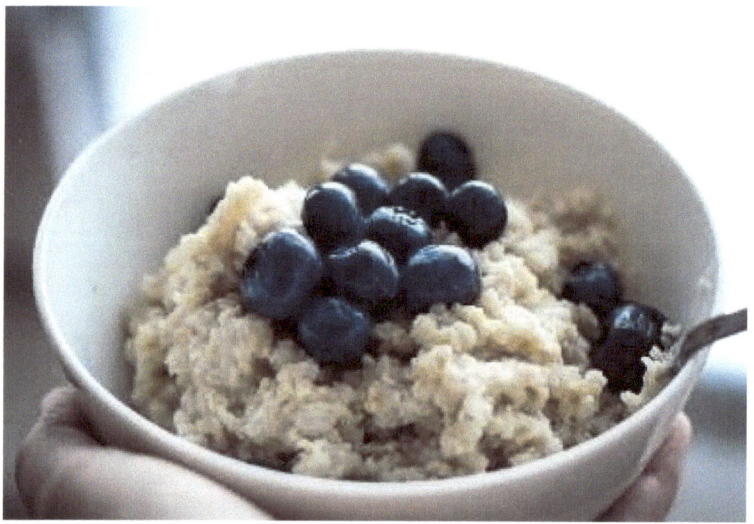

When we're young, we often sabotage our youthful energy by eating the wrong foods. Pizza and hamburgers, laden with high amounts of calories and harmful fats, are often the main diet of children and teens, but may not affect their overall health until they age.

One reason our youthful energy fails as we age is because we're still stuck to the diet of our youth. Pizza, hamburgers and sugary desserts no longer provide our bodies with the types of fuel we need to power the body responsibly.

Eating the wrong foods at any age can zap your energy levels and cause health problems that will plague you throughout your life. The wrong foods may also affect your brain function and motor skills, putting you at high risk for health problems that adversely affect the aging process.

Here are some foods you should eat daily – no matter what age – to help you get through the day and to ensure you have enough energy to do all the things you want to do:

Blueberries – Blueberries on healthy cereal or yogurt or alone as a snack helps to provide oxygen to the brain and establish a healthy balance of vitamins, antioxidants and minerals.

Oatmeal – The combination of oatmeal and fresh blueberries can lower bad cholesterol and help you maintain energy during the day. Whole grain foods digest slowly and provide energy for longer periods of time.

Sweet Potatoes – Studies show that sweet potatoes help slow the aging process and also fight cancer. This high-fiber food can be cooked various ways, including baked and boiled.

Broccoli – Chocked full of micronutrients such as iron, calcium and magnesium and vitamins such as A and C, broccoli helps to fight cancer and can be eaten raw or cooked.

Avocado – This food source contains healthy fats that can help you avoid saturated fats, which are bad for you. Avocados are also a great source of omega-3 fatty acids.

Green Tea – The more we discover about green tea, the more we know it's not only a great antioxidant, but may also be helpful in treating arthritis by diminishing the breakdown of cartilage and reducing inflammation.

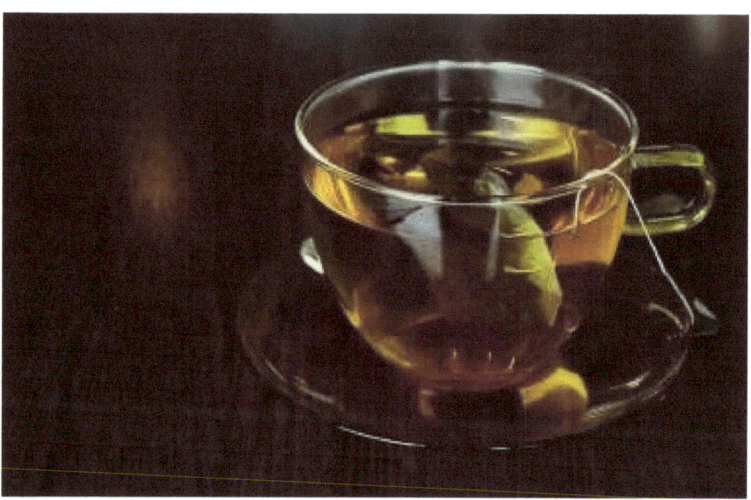

Spinach – Eat fresh spinach whenever you can. It's full of folic acid, which contains vitamin B.

These so-called power foods, plus a few others such as fruits, nuts and some fish can keep up your energy levels during the day, help you get a good night's sleep and ward off the signs of aging.

Energize your mind and body in ways that provide the best nutrition and workouts that bring oxygen to the brain. It's one of the best way to prevent early aging and to enhance your quality of life.

Adopt a Good Beauty and Skincare Regimen

When most people hear the words "anti-aging," they immediately think of wrinkles and how our physical appearance suffers over the years as we age. So let's begin here where we can address the most pressing issue for most men and women.

Beauty is more than just wrinkles – it's how we look head to toe, how we present ourselves aesthetically. Four main areas of your beauty regimen should be in regards to your clothing, your hair, your skincare, and your makeup.

Wear Clothes That Are Age Appropriate

There are many people who will champion your right to wear whatever you want, whenever you want – at any age. And that *is* something to cheer on for those who feel confident enough and happy enough to do that.

But for many others, they desperately *want* to look youthful without embarrassing themselves or making themselves look like they're trying too hard to regain their youth.

If you've always been involved in trends when it comes to clothing, just make sure you evolve your tastes with your age group. Don't try wearing what tweens are wearing if you're 48 years old – no matter how good your body is.

There's more to looking beautiful at any age than being able to show off your midriff or legs. It's about looking elegant and poised in any situation, reflecting confidence and maturity – whether you're 16 or 60.

Don't try to fit in clothes that are too small for you, simply because you've "always been a size 10." You might not be now – as you grow older. A more flattering look would be something that fits your body as you age.

 The older you get, the more sophisticated your look will become. This is a time in your life when you have more stability and more expendable cash than you had in your young twenties, when you shopped on a budget.

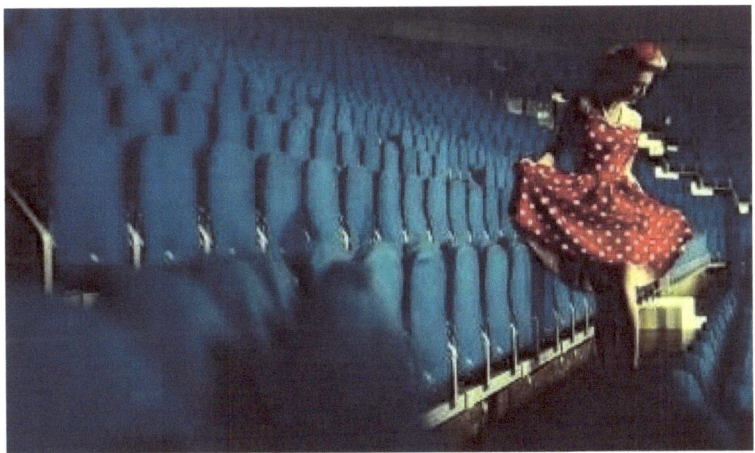

You want to be more aware of matching your outfit with your handbags and shoes. This doesn't mean you have to say goodbye to certain colors – or even certain styles.

You can adapt your tastes as you age so that you're still looking fabulous, but you're not looking like someone who is desperately trying to regain his or her youth through styles or even articles of clothing.

Wear a Hairstyle That Suits Your Age

As we grow older, it becomes more important to take the time needed to get a flattering, age appropriate cut for yourself. There are some people who say there should be no restrictions on hair length in regards to age. In a perfect world…but it's not.

And nobody is telling you that you *have* to get your locks chopped off. But in most cases, whenever you see a makeover show for someone middle aged and beyond, it's the haircut that really shaves years off their look.

The first thing you should know is that as you age, your soft, luscious hair will become wirier and less smooth. It might be curly when it had previously always been straight, or vice versa.

You'll want to adopt a hair regimen that helps condition your strands so that they stay tame in all kinds of weather throughout the day and evening hours when you want it under control.

Second, you'll want to address the color issue. If you're not fond of going gray, you don't have to! You can have your hair colored professionally and simply touch up the roots whenever they grow out.

If these treatments are too expensive, you have options! There are root touchup kits where you simply use what resembles mascara (only for hair) on your roots. You can touch up the part or around your face with it and it washes right out, but blends in until you can afford your next treatment.

Your hairstyle becomes more of a reflection of your personality when you leave trends behind in your teens and twenties and move into your thirties. But in your forties, you have to start weighing whether or not your cut makes you look younger or older.

It's a misconception to believe that the actual cut itself brings about a youthful appeal to you. In reality, a young style might contrast with the rest of you, which is aging, and make you look older.

Some women in their forties will be able to handle any cut. Some won't. It's best to ask your stylist what he or she thinks is fitting for you. You can even have some salons show you digitally what you would look like with a new style.

As you grow older, your hair might thin out, and your cut can be styled to mask the loss of hair to some degree. You want something low maintenance, too – not a style that takes an hour to dry and curl.

Update Your Makeup to Reflect Your Years

Makeup is something that can enhance your natural beauty or hide it and make you look older than your years. You may have enjoyed that when you were 15 trying to look 20, but when you're 40, you want to turn *back* the clock!

Start with your foundation. You probably used a more matte finish in your younger years. This was great if you had oily skin, but as you age, your skin dries out and matte finishes simply showcase fine lines and make you look older.

It will be hard to get used to at first, but try a more sheer makeup with a dewy look – it will make you appear more fresh-faced. You can get one with built in sunscreen to protect your skin.

Forego powder on top of your foundation as you get older. This simply clumps up in your fine lines around your eyes and lips and makes you look harsh – just as the matte foundation does.

When it comes to your eyes, try to make it look as natural as possible when you use eyeliner. Don't use harsh black liner all the way around your eyes – let the club hopping 18-year olds go for that look.

Your eye shadow shouldn't be shimmery or glittery. Keep it natural with muted colors that simply accentuate your eye color, not overpower it. You may need a mascara with more volume if your eyelashes are thinning out.

For your blush, again, avoid hard colors on your cheeks. Now isn't the time to create a hardline streak on your cheekbone like you did when you were younger. Apply it to the apples of your cheeks to help plump up your face – which is especially important if it appears saggy.

On your lips, try to avoid bright colors like blood red. Keep it natural and use a muted color with gloss on your lips. You can still use a lip liner to make your lips appear fuller if you notice they look thinner than before.

Assume a Skincare Regimen Meant for Your Age Group

As you grow older, your skin changes from a tight, flawless appearance to a lined, sagging splotchy look – if you're not careful in preventing and reversing the effects age has on your skin.

At all ages, you should be adhering to a strict sunscreen regimen. It should be applied vigorously anytime you're in the sun for long periods of time, but you can also choose foundation that has SPF in it to protect you throughout your regular daily activities.

In addition to sunscreen, moisturizer should be a staple in your skincare regimen. The more dried out your skin looks, the older you appear to be.

So you want to use daytime creams under your makeup and night creams when you go to bed while your body conducts cellular repair.

You should be using an eye moisturizer that's lighter than the thicker creams you'll be using on the rest of your face. And don't forget about your neck, hands, arms, and the rest of your body.

Don't use skincare products that are full of alcohol, such as toner. This dries your skin out even more. You want to address the hydration issue above all else. Acne might be a problem, but you can spot treat that instead of using an all over treatment.

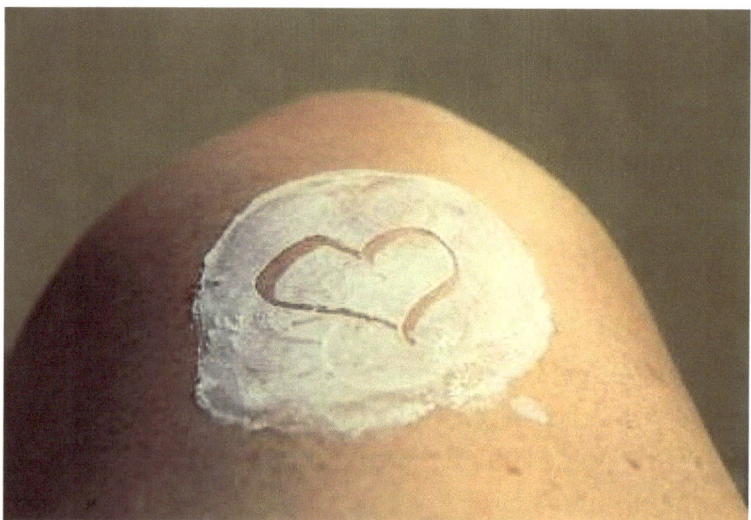

When you exfoliate, it can do two things – remove dead skin cells, which is a benefit, but it can also dry your skin out and cause more harm than good. If you use an exfoliant, use it sparingly – not daily.

Some experts recommend using a retinoid cream at night in lieu of an exfoliant because it helps your body naturally slough off dead skin cells. You wake up with a refreshed look, rather than one that's tired and older in appearance.

Of course, there are more extreme measures you can take, such as getting a chemical peel once a month to remove the topical dead layer of skin cells that age you.

Don't use harsh brushes or pads on your face as you get older. This can damage your delicate skin and it can actually be painful afterwards. Use gentle strokes and avoid pulling on your skin, especially around the eyes.

Never go to sleep with your makeup on. The makeup gets caked into your lines and it prevents your skin from breathing properly, which will inhibit the needed cellular repair.

The truth is, beauty *is* only skin deep. But if you're not taking care of your skin and paying attention to your beauty needs, you'll feel older in years and become depressed about your appearance. It's an easy fix and you should start seeing results right away!

Watching Your Weight as You Grow Older

Studies show that we steadily gain weight as we age. In fact, adults put on an average of nearly one pound per year and most of that gain is caused by changes in our diet.

Extra servings of foods we like can be a big factor in weight gain as we age and we tend to decrease the intake of good foods such as fruits and vegetables. Watching television takes up too much of our time and we don't sleep as well as we did when we were younger.

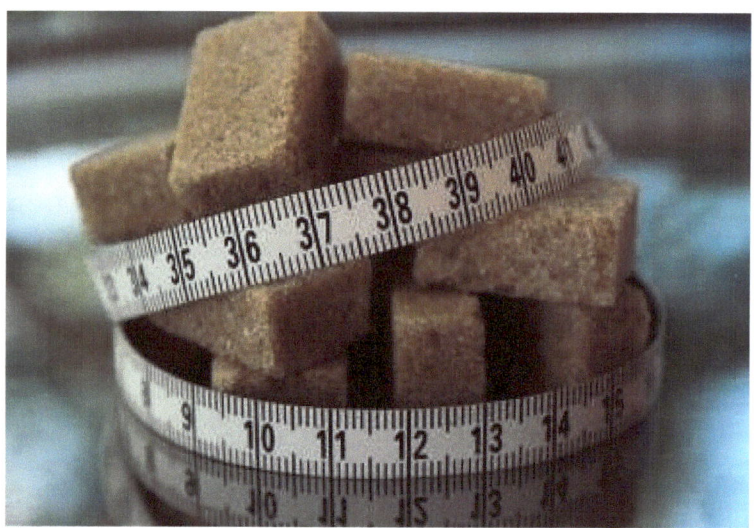

So, dietary and lifestyle choices tend to be the main reasons why we gain weight as we age. As we age it becomes more important to maintain a healthy weight – and that can only be accomplished by adapting a healthy lifestyle.

The Importance of Maintaining a Healthy Weight as We Age

Many experts use your BMI (Body Mass Index) to determine what your ideal weight is based on your height, age and gender. It usually only varies by a pound or so and the National Heart, Lung and Blood Institute states it can be used to determine how healthy you are.

Calculation tools can be readily found on the internet; search for "BMI calculator", enter your details and the tool will calculate your ideal weight. Alternatively, you can calculate it yourself using the following formula:

- Multiply 703 x (present weight).
- Divide that number by your height (inches).
- Divide that number by your height again.

That number will total your BMI. For example 703 x 150lbs./65ins/65ins.=24.9.

A healthy BMI exists within a range, it is not a specific number. The BMI for older women should range between 18.5 and 24.9 (according to the organization 'Livestrong.com'). If you're over the age of 50 and your BMI is between 25 and 30, you're in the overweight category. If it's over 30, you are considered obese.

Obesity can have a harmful impact on your health as you age, so it becomes very important to eat well – especially during the ages when your metabolism is slowing down and you may not be as active as in your youth.

How to Increase Your Metabolism as You Age

It's a fact that our metabolism slows down as we age. There's nothing we can do about 'mother nature', but we can take steps to help keep our bodies working enough to keep off extra weight.

We don't always notice a slowing metabolism. There are no real changes that we experience except a pound or two that creeps on and our clothes may not fit right.

As we age, our physical activity lessens, our hormonal balance changes and this causes our muscle mass to decrease. At the same time and for the same reasons, the body begins to lay down a layer of fat. We may be eating about the same amount as always, but with a slowing metabolism, we're not burning as many calories as we take in. The body naturally stores this excess as fat.

Besides a slowing metabolism, we're also affected by less manufacturing of the human growth hormone that builds and maintains muscle mass. Muscle burns calories and if our muscle mass diminishes, it becomes more difficult to burn off the fat.

Keeping the metabolism functioning at its ultimate pace only requires three simple steps:

Healthy Lifestyle – Simply stated, a healthy lifestyle means giving up the bad habits such as smoking, drinking too much alcohol and consuming calorie-laden, high-GI foods.

Healthy Diet – Adding fruits, vegetables, whole grains and other foods that promote health rather than detract from it is one way to increase or maintain a high-functioning metabolism.

Exercise – This step is critical in maintaining a healthy weight and keeping the metabolism purring even as we age. A good exercise program that includes some aerobics, muscle building and stretching is one of the best things we can do for our wellbeing and longevity.

Your metabolism plays a huge part in keeping you healthy and keeping your weight in check. Do everything you can as you age to ensure that your metabolism will work at its best during your older years.

Avoiding the Traps of Weight Gain as You Age

Don't think at all that weight gain is inevitable as you age. You may not be as peppy as you were as a teenager or during the height of your working years, but you don't have to be stuck with extra weight that makes you unhealthy and keeps you from enjoying life.

Avoiding weight gain as you age may be as simple as replacing the old foods that you used to love – like French fries and hamburgers – with healthier and less calorie laden foods such as fruits and vegetables.

Here are some traps that might carry on from younger years, when we can easier maintain an ideal weight – to older years when it may not be so easy:

Adhering to the "Modern" Diet of Simple Carbohydrates and Sugars – One trap of putting on weight as we age is to maintain the diet we had when we were young, and think we can still get away with it!

If your diet has regular inclusions of sweets, cakes, desserts after meals and between meal treats you will struggle to maintain a healthy weight. In addition, you will have erratic blood glucose levels and will be subjecting your system to excessive insulin releases. This will affect the health of organs such as your liver and pancreas and risk contracting Type 2 diabetes.

Insufficient Exercise – As we age, some of the muscle mass we had when we were young diminishes and is replaced by fat.

To fight this phenomenon of aging, exercise that is designed to build and maintain muscle is imperative. Also, maintaining an active, aerobic lifestyle to keep up our metabolism can help keep the muscle we have and convert body fat to needed energy.

Genetics Role in Obesity as We Age – Our relatives play an important role in our weight gain as we age. If our mothers and grandmothers were naturally slim, changes are we will too.

Don't give up if your genetics aren't what you'd like them to be. Consider your genetic makeup a 'predisposition' only; your actions still play a major role in your body shape and overall health. You can still pare down the weight by living a super-healthy lifestyle, getting plenty of exercise and not giving in to the fate that life seems to have given you.

The 'Couch Potato' Trap – While we may not feel like running a marathon as we age, it is not in the best interest of our physical, mental or emotional health to give in to the trap of spending our evenings on the couch watching mindless television programs.

Get up and move! Walk around the block, take up a hobby or take a class at the local college. Not only will moving help activate your slowing metabolism – it will also help stave off the mental effects of aging.

Beware of the traps that can add weight to your body. Keeping a healthy body and mind are keys to remaining young at heart and feeling good about yourself. Don't strive for that bikini body you had when you were 16, but find out what's normal for you and put in the effort to stay as healthy as you can be at whatever age you are at. Your health will be you reward.

Final Thoughts

There is no doubt that dealing with some aspects of aging require great effort. However, it should also be acknowledged that maturity also brings some respite from many of the concerns and problems that challenged us when we were younger.

We should all have the right to age happily, without fear or dread. We should also accept responsibility for as much autonomous action as we are able, so that we can be as empowered as our circumstances allow.

Dealing with changes to our bodies, our environments, lifestyles and technologies with a healthy mindset will allow us to enjoy growing older instead of resenting it. Love your life.

Other Relevant Books by This Author

If you would like to read more about health and fitness for seniors, here is a list of the CreateSpace links, titles and brief descriptions:

https://www.createspace.com/4963196

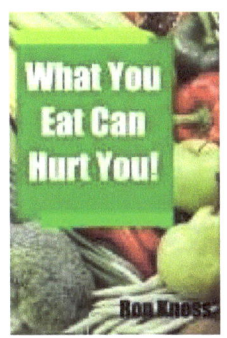

What You Eat Can Hurt You

Do you know that certain foods increase your risk for inflammation, disease and illness? It's true! And certain foods can help cure and heal you if you do get sick. Knowing which foods to eat and which ones to avoid empowers you to manage your own health.

https://www.createspace.com/4962939

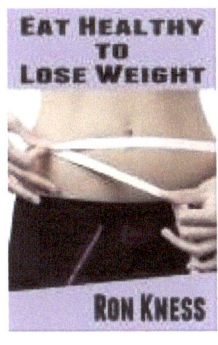

Eat Healthy to Lose Weight

As you read through our book, we show you which foods you should and should not be eating to reach your weight loss goal, along with discussing how to maintain your weight loss and stay within a few pounds of your goal weight. Banish the weight you keep gaining back each time by learning how to live a healthy lifestyle.

https://www.createspace.com/5252272

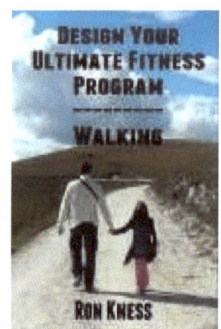

Design Your Ultimate Fitness Program - Walking

In my book Design Your Ultimate Fitness Program – Walking, we discuss the considerations that need to be made when designing a custom walking program, along with:

• Equipment needed

• Wearable technology you can use to track your walking

• And how to make walking more challenging

https://www.createspace.com/5474751

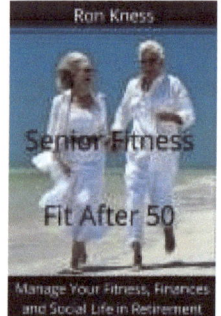

Senior Fitness – Fit After 50: Learn How to Manage Your Fitness, Finances and Social Life in Retirement

Inside you will discover answers to your most pressing questions:

• What do I need to know about downsizing my home?

• What are the best tips for staying healthy as you approach your 50's?

• When should I start planning for retirement?

• I am worried about being lonely once I retire, do others feel the same?

• Is it worthwhile to carry two homes during retirement?

And more…

https://www.createspace.com/6299671

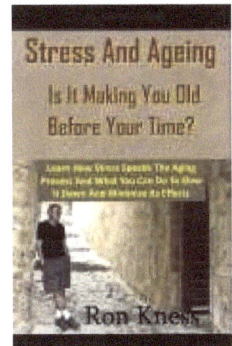

Stress and Ageing – Is It Making You Old Before Your Time?
The stress response occurs when external or internal factors cause the body's adrenal glands to put out excess epinephrine, norepinephrine, and cortisol.

These response hormones can result in an increased heart rate, respiratory rate, blood pressure, and blood glucose levels.

A stressor can be anything from having a bad day at the office, relationship issues, physical or emotional distress, financial problems, and a whole host of other things that infiltrate our daily lives, resulting in a stress response.

While stress is normal, too much of it, or too often, can lead to negative effects on your health. In this book we discuss how to recognize stress and how to minimize its effects to keep you from getting old before your time.

https://www.createspace.com/5404845

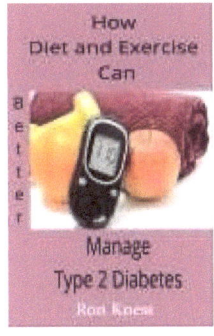

How Diet and Exercise Can Better Manage Type 2 Diabetes
Of the different types of diabetes, only Type 2 can be reversed. In my book How Diet and Exercise Can Better Manage Type 2 Diabetes, we reveal the three things you can do to best manage your disease, including:
• Diet

- Exercise
- Weight management

https://www.createspace.com/5464020

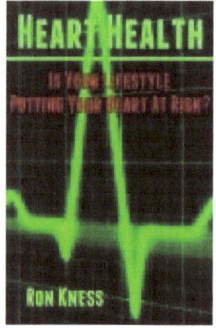

Heart Health: Is Your Lifestyle Putting Your Heart at Risk?
In my ebook Is Your Lifestyle Putting Your Heart At Risk? we discuss the six greatest risks to your heart and the lifestyle changes you can make to mitigate them.

https://www.createspace.com/5457441

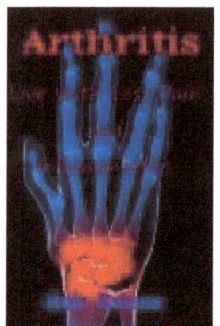

Arthritis – Live Wth Less Pain and Inflammation: Tips and Techniques You Can Use to Lessen the Pain and Inflammation
Discover Simple Tips & Information That Will Help Reduce The Painful Symptoms Of Arthritis!

You learn things like:
- Simple and effective information that will help you manage the pain and inflammation that comes along with arthritis, so that you can live an active, full life without debilitating pain.
- The different types of arthritis, their symptoms and how to alleviate their painful side effects.
- The pros and cons of over-the-counter arthritis medications, plus simple tips that will help you know how to choose the right supplements.
- Free, yet effective ways to get relief from arthritis pain and inflammation, so you don't have to suffer anymore.

The effects arthritis can have significant impact on your physical and mental well-being, but this books shows you how to overcome its painful symptoms and live life relatively pain free.

https://www.createspace.com/6737019

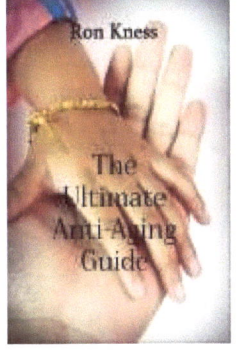

The Ultimate Anti-Aging Guide
Discover the techniques and methods to reverse the aging process so you can look and feel younger.

What you'll discover in this book:
- How aging works and why your skin changes
- The difference between the products currently available
- How to combine different types of products for maximal results
- Why exercise and mindset it so important
- How to change a few things for HUGE results
- How to keep your hair young and strong for longer
- How to prevent your hands from getting old
- How to stop age showing on your face
- How to work out
- How to treat common aging problems
- ...and much, much more!

Nobody likes getting (or looking) old. However, there are many things you can do to look younger than your actual age. Why not try them! What you have to lose besides looking years younger.

https://www.createspace.com/5416348

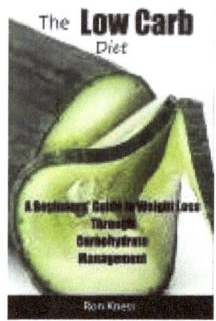

The Low Carb Diet: A Beginner's Guide to Weight Loss Through Carbohydrate Management

In my book "The Low-Carb Diet – A Beginners' Guide to Weight Loss Through Carbohydrate Management", I reveal a successful method of losing weight based in part on the amount and type of carbohydrates you consume.

https://www.createspace.com/5714434

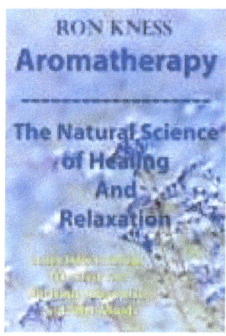

Aromatherapy - The Science of Healing and Relaxation: Learn How Essential Oils Elicit The Relaxation Response And Alter Mood

In my book Aromatherapy – The Science of Healing and Relaxation, we reveal the natural holistics methods you can use to heal the body from certain medical issues and to relive stress through relaxation. In particular we talk about:

• Aromatherapy - what it is and how it works

• Essential Oils – how the effects of certain aromas differs from others

• Recipes – how to make your own essential oil combinations

About the Author

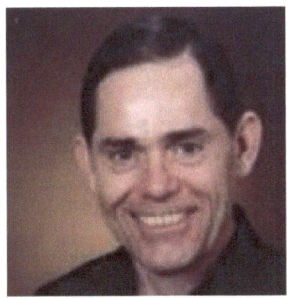

I grew up in Central Minnesota, where my parents owned and operated a fishing resort. Once out of high school I tried a couple of semesters of college, only to quit halfway through the Spring term; I decided at that time that college wasn't for me.

Then I decided to follow my father's previous occupation as an auto mechanic. I graduated from a two-year of vocational training course and worked as a mechanic for five years. While in vocational training, I decided to join the National Guard where I eventually ended up working full-time for 32 years.

So how does all of this relate to writing? In one of my leadership schools, the instructor, who was an English teacher at a juvenile detention center, presented writing to me in a whole new way - a way that started to develop my interest in working with words.

I eventually went back to college on the GI Bill while I was working and earned my Bachelor's degree in Business Administration.

Taking a class or two per semester at night and on weekends took me seven years to complete my degree.

Fast forward about 40 years and I now have published over 100 books on Amazon for Kindle, CreateSpace and other publishing platforms.

Besides my own writing, I also ghostwrite ebooks, books, reports, articles, blogs and do Kindle conversions for clients on a variety of topics.

Today my wife and I are retired from our careers and live in Gold Canyon, AZ. I now write as a retirement business where you'll find me happily sitting in my office typing away on my laptop as I work on my next book or ghostwriting project . . . that is if we are not traveling on a cruise ship - our new-found mode of travel.